# FOOD

Simple Ways to Nourish
Your Body and Soul

# FOR

# THOUGHT

Written and Illustrated By

## Julianne Kanzaki

MPH, RDN, NBC-HWC

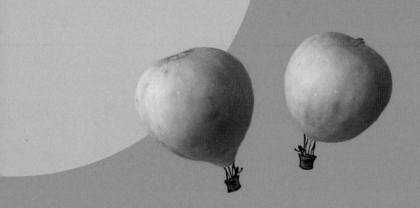

# PRAISE *for*
# FOOD FOR
# THOUGHT

"On behalf of the plants of the world, I offer gratitude to Julianne Kanzaki for giving voice to the endless ways that plants delight the spirit, inspire creativity, and evoke vitality. Julianne brilliantly celebrates plants not only for their bodily healing qualities, but for how they nourish our deeper social, emotional, and spiritual well-being."

**KATE VOGT,** author of *Our Inherited Wisdom* and co-editor of *Mala of Love* and *Mala of the Heart*

"I can brazenly declare that the only thing I've loved longer than written words — family not included — is food, and never have I seen the two brought together in such an engaging, thoughtful, and nourishing way as they have been in *Food For Thought*. However, nowhere in this delicious, appetite-inducing book of food wisdom does Julianne call herself a poet, but she is that, undoubtedly!"

**DARNELL LAMONT WALKER,** Emmy Nominated Children's Media Writer

"Julianne's creativity and artistry inspire and educate. In her unique style, she has packed this book with incredible art, fun facts, and nutritional advice to jumpstart your journey into health and well-being."

**STEPHEN EZEJI-OKOYE,** MD

"*Food For Thought* is packed with incredible information and fun facts, and it also weaves deeper, empowering messages throughout. Reading alongside my four children, giggles grew with anticipation, as each food illustration greeted us with creativity and whimsy page after page. Already we have used the wisdom and guidance in this book to set some personal and food goals — picking out some new things to try from our favorite pages using the practical tips included. Whether you are five or 95, you'll learn something new — definitely about food, but maybe even something about yourself, too."

**NADINE FONSECA,** CEO at Mighty Kind, author of *Only a Trenza Away*

Published by Julianne Kanzaki
juliannekanzaki.com

ISBN 9798858600725
Library of Congress Control Number: 2023919384

Cover Art: Julianne Kanzaki
Cover and Book Design: Matthew Meikle

This book is dedicated to

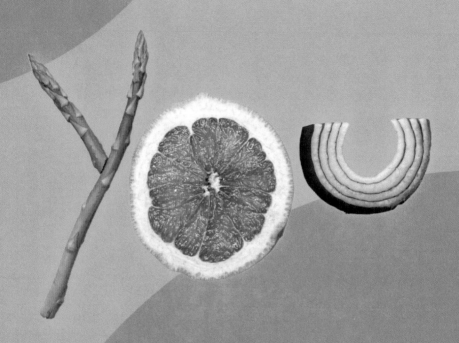

and the unique way you see
and contribute to the world.

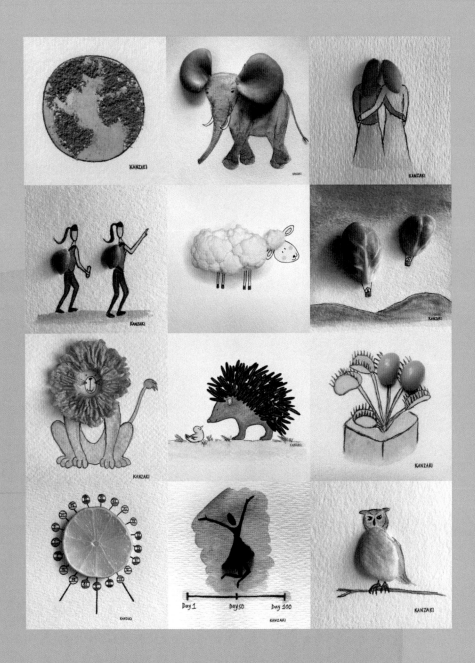

Dear Reader,

Sometimes the best things in life are made organically out of pure joy.

The book you're holding is one such creation. It began as a personal art project where I made food illustrations for 100 days.

During this time, I paid closer attention as I cut mushrooms, washed broccoli crowns, and harvested herbs. Through this creative lens, I was inspired by the endless possibilities that existed when I slowed down to notice them.

I realized the ordinary has the power to become extraordinary.

As a dietitian, I'm delighted to share vibrant whole foods that can support your health. But more importantly, I hope these pages encourage you to free your imagination. See your environment from a refreshingly new perspective. Awaken to the magic that is all around you.

Peas and Love,

Julianne

# TABLE OF CONTENTS

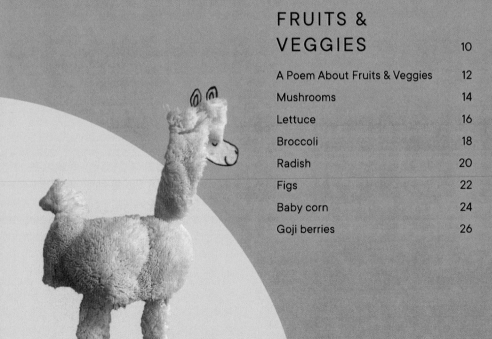

# FRUITS & VEGGIES

# FRUITS & VEGGIES

## MUSHROOMS

## LETTUCE

## BROCCOLI

## RADISH

## FIGS

## BABY CORN

## GOJI BERRIES

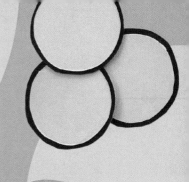

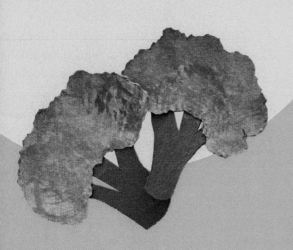

A POEM ABOUT

# FRUITS & VEGGIES

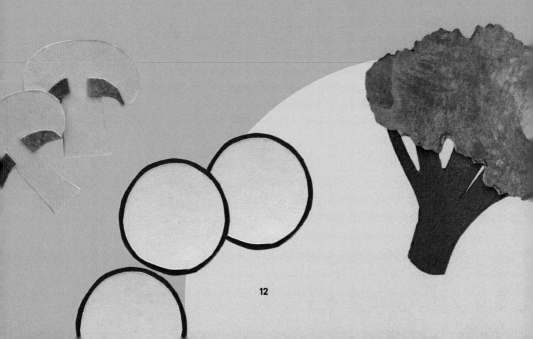

Fruits and vegetables provide nutrients
to play, jump, and run.
Growing them ourselves
makes eating them more fun!

Fertilize the soil,
then gently plant the seeds.
Give them time, sun, and water,
simple are their needs.

Nature IS our nature,
and when we're connected to our food,
we're supported in a deeper way
that uplifts our mood.

Each one of their colors
provides antioxidants only found
in that particular produce,
so eat the rainbow all around!

Diversity is key
and it's always much more fun
when our plates are full of color
radiating energy from the sun.

Start first with ones you like,
then keep adding something new.
Continue to experiment —
there's 300,000 from to choose!

When we nourish our bodies
with fruits and veggies that are real,
it positively changes
the way we think and feel.

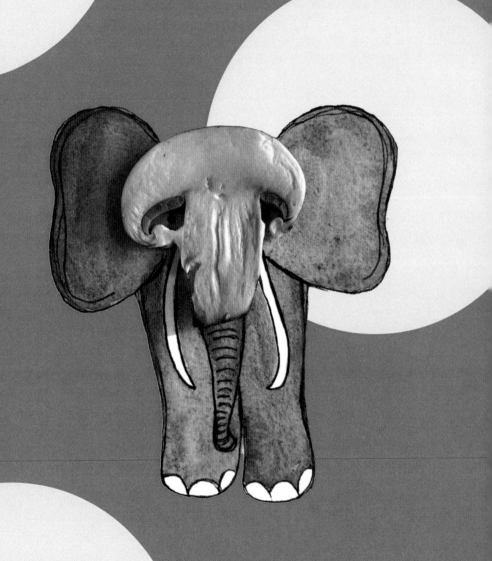

# MUSHROOMS

Elephants teach us how there's so MUSHROOM for improvement in the current ways we lead and serve in our communities.

Elephants model how gentleness, commitment, and clear communication build trusting and loving relationships. The matriarch is fiercely protective, yet she leads in a way that is both gentle and inclusive. How can you also lead in nurturing and loving ways within your community?

**FUN FACTS**

Button, cremini, and portobello mushrooms are the same mushroom species, *Agaricus bisporus*. The only difference is their age. Button mushrooms are the youngest. Cremini mushrooms have brown caps and no visible gills. They are harvested later than button mushrooms. Portobellos are mature *Agaricus bisporus*. Mushrooms are technically fungi and contain B vitamins and prebiotics, which fight inflammation, improve cognition, and help balance and support our immune system.

---

**WAYS TO ENJOY**

Add porcini, chanterelle, or oyster mushrooms to pasta or pizza, or include shiitake to soups and stir-fries to add umami flavor. Grill portobello mushrooms for a delicious and nutrient-dense burger alternative.

# LETTUCE

LETTUCE be aware of our thoughts and environment. Are you swimming in self-doubt, anxiety, and fear? Or self-compassion, curiosity, and acceptance?

Notice the emotions and attitudes of the people closest to you. Energy is contagious. Monitor what you read, watch, and listen to. Every input positively or negatively affects how you think and feel. Make a conscious effort to swim in an environment that best supports your mental and physical health.

**FUN FACTS**

The first Roman emperor, Augustus Caesar, constructed a statue to honor romaine lettuce. When he was seriously ill and traditional medications failed to work, he believed his diet, which largely consisted of romaine lettuce, cured him. Another type of lettuce, iceberg, got its name in 1920 when California growers began shipping it covered with crushed ice. Before this, it was called Crisphead lettuce.

Compared to iceberg lettuce, romaine lettuce contains twice as much Vitamin A, supporting healthy eyesight. In addition, it has four times as much Vitamin K, which aids in bone health, and 75% more fiber, which promotes smooth digestion.

**WAYS TO ENJOY**

The next time you choose lettuce, skip the iceberg and create a diverse blend by mixing romaine, arugula, spinach, kale, frisée, and radicchio for a colorful, vibrant, and nutritious salad base.

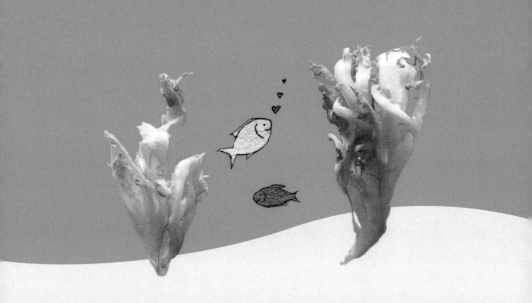

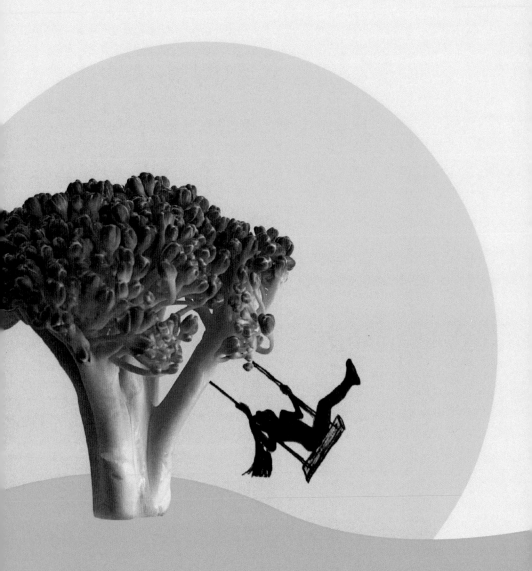

# BROCCOLI

If you're working on a task and feel stuck, it's time to play! So step away, switch to a more enjoyable activity, ideally head outside, and most of all, have fun.

When you return to your original task, you'll feel refreshed. Creativity expands when we loosen up. You may find a new solution to an old problem or discover a novel connection you hadn't yet seen.

The next time you hit a wall mentally or creatively, get some fresh air, move your body, and play!

**FUN FACTS**

One cup of broccoli contains 3g of protein and sulforaphane, a potent anti-cancer and anti-inflammatory phytochemical. But, more impressively, broccoli sprouts contain over 100 times the amount of sulforaphane than mature broccoli.

---

**WAYS TO ENJOY**

Add steamed or roasted broccoli to stir-fries and pasta, or julienne broccoli stalks for broccoli slaw. You can start sprouting broccoli at home. All you need is a mason jar, cheesecloth, and broccoli seeds. When they sprout within a few days, sprinkle them on salads and add them to wraps for added texture and nutrition.

# RADISH

You may think you need an expensive or RADISH-looking triathlon bike to participate in the sport. But truthfully, all you need is an open mind and a basic bike, swimsuit, and running shoes.

For my first sprint triathlon, I used a road bike that didn't have clip-in pedals. I didn't know how to properly shift gears, so I rode the entire bike portion in the same gear. I successfully finished and had so much fun that I decided to push myself further and sign up for another race. Little did I know, this was the start of my Ironman journey.

We often assume we need the best equipment to begin our health journey. The reality is that we just need to start.

**FUN FACTS**

In November 2020, NASA astronaut Kate Rubins harvested fresh radishes grown in the Advanced Plant Habitat (APH) aboard the International Space Station. As a result, new doors are opening now for producing food in microgravity to sustain future longer-term missions in space.

**WAYS TO ENJOY**

The roots, leaves, and seeds of the radish are all edible. Add colorful red globe or watermelon radishes to salads and slaws, or enjoy pickled daikon radish as a side dish or in Bahn mi sandwiches.

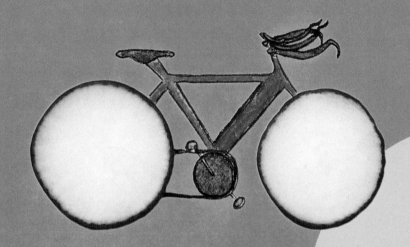

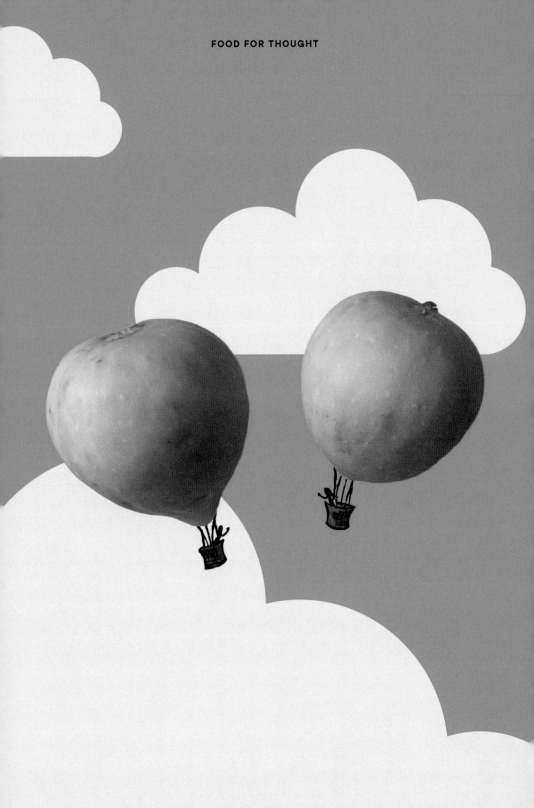

# FIGS

## Even if you don't have everything FIGured out in life, you can still uplift others on their journey.

You are brave. You are resilient. You've been knocked down and have gotten back up. Maybe you've had your heart broken but chose to love again. Perhaps you've switched jobs or started a family. Maybe you decided not to start a family. Maybe you finally realized that your purpose is not defined by what you do but by who you are. Keep showing up. You never know how your story is silently encouraging and inspiring someone else.

**FUN FACTS**

Figs need fig wasps to pollinate. Their relationship is unique because each needs the other to complete its life cycle. A female wasp first bores into a fig. Then, she moves from flower to flower, laying eggs and spreading the pollen she brought with her from the fig where she was born. This is her one crucial mission. Afterward, she dies, and fig trees produce an enzyme called fican, which dissolves her body. These nutrients are then used to nourish the fig. When the larvae hatch, the male larvae mate with the females. Later, the mature female wasps exit and visit other figs, delivering pollen from the previous fig to complete the life cycle.

**WAYS TO ENJOY**

Figs taste delicious raw, grilled on a pizza, as a jam, mixed with salads, or stuffed with nuts and cheese for a sweet and savory flavor combination.

# BABY CORN

May these words remind you
in case you forgot,
When life feels heavy
because you're juggling a lot...

There's no one like you
with your gifts and your heart,
Your smile, perspective,
your humor and art!

The world became brighter
the day you were born
You're powerful! You're magical!
You are a uni-CORN!

**FUN FACTS**

Another name for baby corn is cornlettes.
Baby corn is harvested early while the stalks
are still immature. Growing and harvesting baby
corn is a labor-intensive process. As soon as the
corn silk begins peeking out, baby corn is hand-
harvested. Nutritionally, baby corn contains
carotenoids and fiber to support healthy eyesight
and regular digestion.

---

**WAYS TO ENJOY**

Add baby corn to stir-fries, soups, curries,
stews, and noodle dishes. Mix baby corn with
lettuce, mandarin oranges, and a ginger sesame
vinaigrette for a refreshing salad combination. In
the mood for something savory? Lightly coat baby
corn with BBQ sauce and air fry at 400 degrees F
for 8–10 minutes for a yummy side dish or snack.

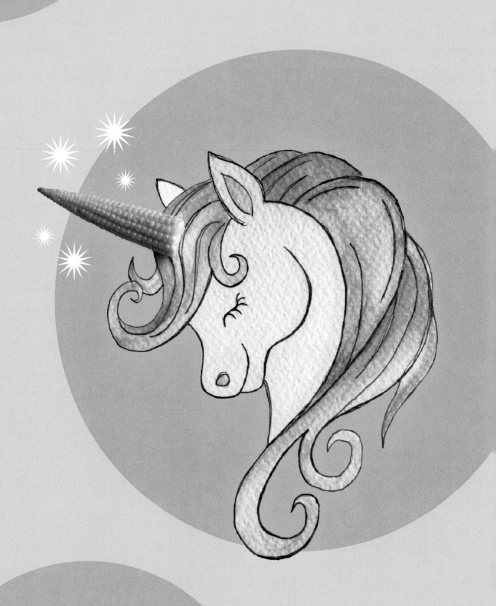

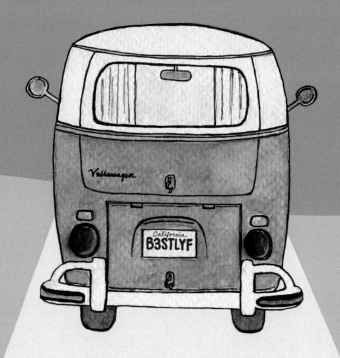

# GOJI BERRIES

On the road of life, travel light. Bring only the essential and meaningful people and things with you.

Spring cleaning isn't just for our physical spaces. Clearing out digital clutter feels just as freeing and cathartic. Remove apps you don't use on your devices. Clear old message threads and update your contacts. Remember, you intentionally control what you invite into your mental and energetic space. Clearing out the old frees up more space to say 'yes' to the people, experiences, and opportunities that best support you moving forward on your path.

**FUN FACTS**

Goji berries boost the immune system, support healthy skin, and protect the eyes. Three tablespoons of dried goji berries provide 3mg or 15% of the recommended daily value for iron. A 1 oz. serving of goji berries contains more Vitamin C than oranges, more beta carotene than carrots, and is full of fiber and antioxidants.

**WAYS TO ENJOY**

Add dried goji berries to baked goods or trail mix, sprinkle over oatmeal, or add as toppings to smoothies or acai bowls. They're also a convenient and delicious antioxidant-rich snack on their own.

# PROTEIN

# PROTEIN

---

PINTO BEANS

---

MUNG BEANS

---

BLACK BEANS

---

CHICKPEAS

## A POEM ABOUT

# PROTEIN

It's a common misconception
that protein only comes from meat.
But plants alone can meet our needs,
isn't that so neat?

There are 20 amino acids,
all are abundantly found in plants.
It's easy to meet your protein needs,
just simply mix and match!

Chickpeas, black beans, and lentils,
tofu, quinoa, and moong dal —
have heart-healthy benefits,
helping to lower cholesterol.

The benefit of plant proteins
is they come wrapped with a gift
of prebiotic fiber
which helps our gut and mind to shift.

So for all you animal lovers,
here's a solution for how to eat
in a way that protects our animals
and the earth beneath our feet.

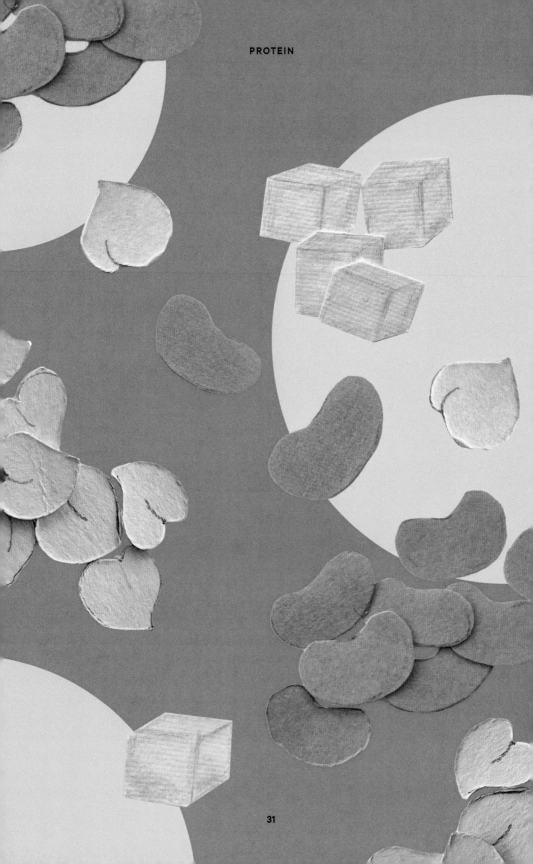

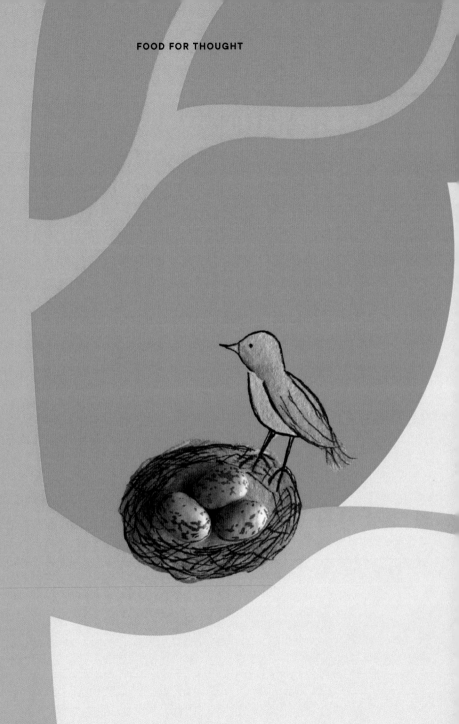

# PINTO BEANS

BEAN patient is a virtue. Everything hatches at the right moment. Learn to be gentle with yourself during any journey, whether you're making changes to eat healthier, move your body more consistently, or taking on a new role at work.

Big successes nor breakthroughs happen overnight. But with consistency and a supportive environment, trust that you will hatch out of your shell at the right time.

| | |
|---|---|
| **FUN FACTS** | Pinto beans are the most popular type of bean consumed in America. In Spanish, "pinto" means painted; visually, pinto beans look like a speckled painting. Nutritionally, one ½ cup serving of pinto beans provides 8g of fiber and 8g of protein. |

| | |
|---|---|
| **WAYS TO ENJOY** | Enjoy pinto beans in a variety of dishes, including chili, burritos, dips, enchiladas, and soups. Add them to fajitas, sautéed veggies, or top them with pickled onions or pico de gallo for a pop of bright color and flavor. |

# MUNG BEANS

Even if you're the slowest aMUNGst your friends, you're perfect just the way you are. Some people need extra time to start (or end) their day, to think about things, and make decisions.

Our brains also have two speeds of thinking. Compared to fast thinking, slow thinking is more deliberate, conscious, and aware. It helps us recognize emotions, pay attention, and considerately respond.

Allow your life to unfold organically on its own timeline, and trust the process. Don't feel pressured to rush or change who you are to match our fast-paced environment. Instead, embrace the beautiful way you're created. The world benefits from how you model slowing down and living more thoughtfully, mindfully, and present.

**FUN FACTS**

Just ¼ cup (dry) of mung beans contains 12g of protein and 8g of fiber. Sprouted mung beans contain higher amounts of antioxidants, helping the body fight off free radicals and prevent chronic disease.

**WAYS TO ENJOY**

Sprouted mung beans can be easily added to stir-fries or sprinkled on top of salads to support a healthy gut microbiome and keep you full, satisfied, and energized.

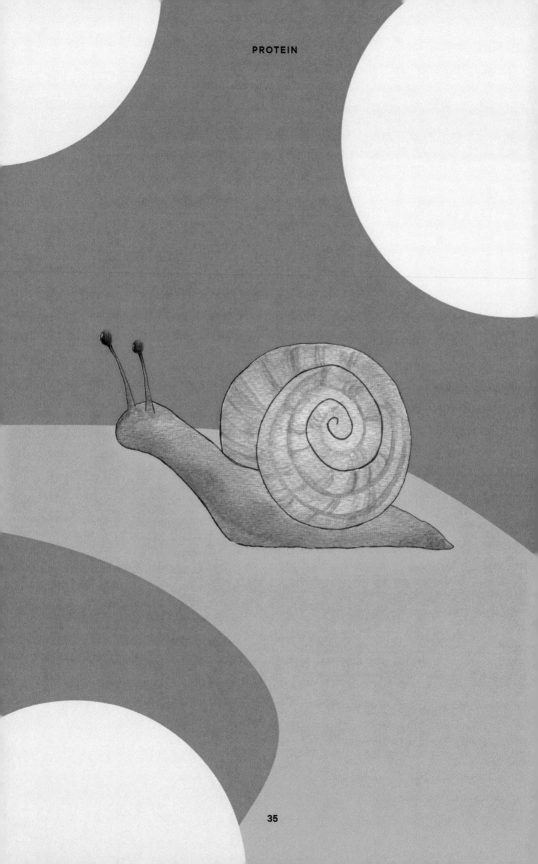

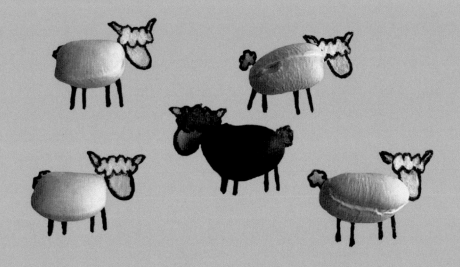

# BLACK BEANS

Just BEAN yourself is the greatest gift you can give the world. There is no one else like you. Your ideas. Your vision. Your skills. You are not meant to fit in. You are meant to stand out!

**FUN FACTS**

Black beans stand out nutritionally because they contain high amounts of antioxidants, help lower blood cholesterol, prevent heart disease, and stabilize blood sugar. One cup of cooked black beans contains 15g of protein and 4.8g of soluble fiber.

---

**WAYS TO ENJOY**

Add them into salads, mix them into burrito bowls or wraps, or enjoy a black bean burger for a nutrient-dense powerhouse of antioxidants, protein, folate, and fiber.

# CHICKPEAS

There was a chapter in my life when I felt broken, lost, and sad. Everything about my future was uncertain. My dad gifted me with the most powerful object lesson during that time. Sitting at the potter's wheel, he held up a piece of clay. "Sometimes the clay doesn't turn out exactly how the potter intended. Does this mean he throws away the clay?"

He paused and gently looked me in the eyes. "No. He doesn't give up on it. He simply re-centers and reshapes it."

I think about this often. Sometimes life — in its lumpy, pathetic, lopsided form — just needs time. Life requires generous amounts of patience and grace and second chances and hope. It needs us to stay humble and malleable. Even if uncomfortable, trust that you are being shaped into something else. Something new and better.

**FUN FACTS**   Chickpea coffee, made from roasted and ground chickpeas, has been around since the 18th century. It's a caffeine-free alternative to coffee and contains antioxidants, folate, magnesium, and fiber for digestion and heart health.

**WAYS TO ENJOY**   There are many ways to appreciate chickpeas aside from hummus and falafel. Roasted chickpeas make the perfect protein and fiber-rich savory and crunchy snack. Add chickpeas to nourish bowls, curries, or soups. Use ground chickpea flour (besan) as the foundation for crepes that you can fill with stir-fried vegetables for a balanced meal. When using canned chickpeas, save the liquid (aquafaba) to make your own dairy-free, nut-free meringue cookies.

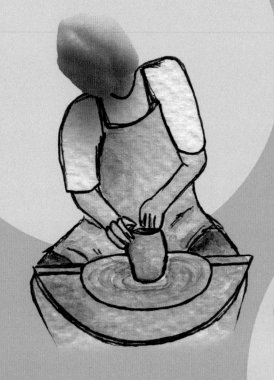
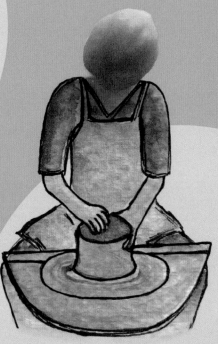

# FATS

A POEM ABOUT

# FATS

---

# WALNUTS

---

# MIXED NUTS
(Cashews, Almonds, Peanuts)

---

# AVOCADO

---

# OLIVES

## A POEM ABOUT

# FATS

Plant fats are nutritious,
like avocados, nuts, and seeds.
They help us to feel satisfied
and contribute to energy needs.

Almond, peanut, and sunbutter
are crowd favorites, that's for sure!
With their rich and creamy texture,
choose the ones you have to stir.

Anti-inflammatory fatty acids
are called omega-3s,
they're not only in fish, they're also in plants
like walnuts and flaxseeds.

Unlike animal fats,
they're naturally cholesterol-free,
supporting heart health, lowering inflammation-
so many benefits for you and me!

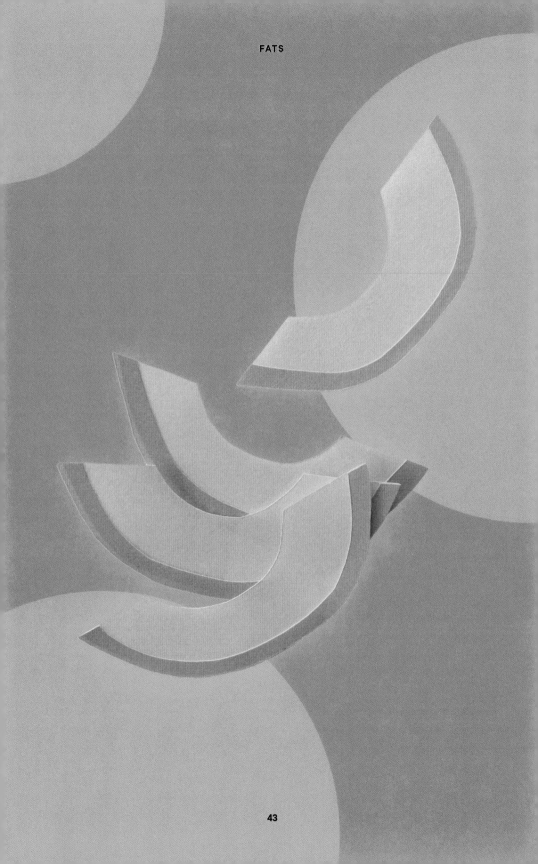

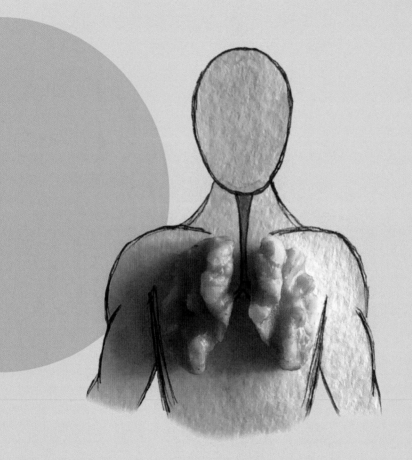

# WALNUTS

One of the fastest ways to decrease stress is by using your breath. The 2:1 breathing technique is a simple and accessible way to help reduce stress on the spot. A quick double inhale, followed by a long, deep exhale, helps calm the nervous system and facilitates relaxation.

'Inspire' comes from the Latin word 'inspirare,' which means 'to breathe into.' As creative human beings, it's important to feel inspired. However, be careful not to spend too much time chasing inspiration that you forget to exhale and make your own art. Instead, balance your inspiration with exhalation. Give and take. Consume and create.

**FUN FACTS**

Walnuts are the oldest tree food known to man, dating back to 7000 B.C. In ancient herbalism, the term "Doctrine of Signatures" refers to how a plant resembles the organ system it supports in the body. Walnuts look like a human brain and contain more omega–3 fatty acids than any other nut. Omega–3 fatty acids promote healthy brain function, memory, and mood.

**WAYS TO ENJOY**

Sprinkle raw or toasted walnuts in your oatmeal and salads for added texture and nutrition. Or, use walnuts to make muhammara, a delicious roasted red pepper dip.

# MIXED NUTS

This may sound NUTS, but if you're interested in RAISIN your vibration, look carefully at the people you surround yourself with. Intentionally spend time with individuals who are optimistic, growth-oriented, and curious.

When measured, positive emotions like joy and gratitude radiate higher vibrational frequencies in comparison to lower frequency emotions like guilt and shame.

Just like nuts are good for heart health, so are good friends. I'm grateful that my friends inspire me to take creative risks, step outside my comfort zone, and encourage me athletically. By leading with these qualities, they enable me to see the world from an abundant, expansive lens.

**FUN FACTS**

Trail mix has been eaten by Native Americans for thousands of years, and their original mix included buffalo meat. Trail mix is also called "GORP," which stands for "Good Old Raisins and Peanuts." According to the Oxford English Dictionary, the word gorp means "to eat greedily."

---

**WAYS TO ENJOY**

Nuts and raisins are ideal snacks for hiking since they are portable and lightweight. Raisins offer a quick energy boost, and the healthy fats in nuts provide sustainable energy to keep your body well-fueled on the trails. In addition, you won't have to worry about them melting in your bag!

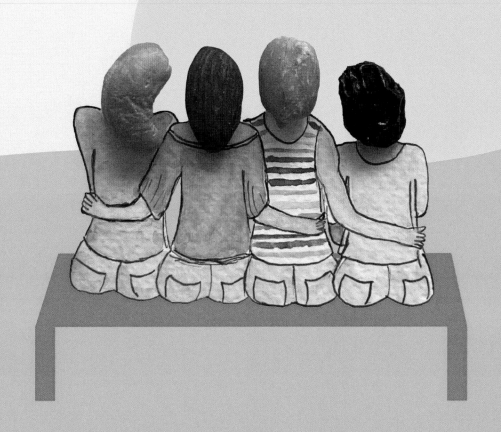

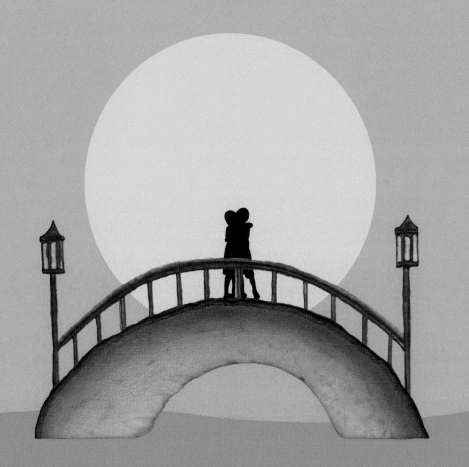

# AVOCADO

We all remember when someone said something hurtful to us. How awful and crushing it felt.

Now think about a time when someone gifted you with a kind and encouraging word. Bask in how empowering, transformative, and uplifting it was. How it made you feel more confident and seen. During some of the most challenging times in my life, I was buoyed by thoughtful and loving words from others.

Recently at a retreat, I was searching for a place to sit when I heard a sweet voice. "You can sit here!" That simple offer was the beginning of a beautiful friendship. Words have power. They can be invitations to connect in deeper, more meaningful ways. Use them to build bridges, not walls.

**FUN FACTS**

Surprisingly, avocados contain more potassium than bananas. A single avocado contains 975mg of potassium, compared to 487mg in a banana. And just one-half of an avocado (100g) boasts 7g fiber! Need to ripen an avocado quickly? Place it in a brown paper bag with bananas. The bananas release ethylene gas, which expedites the ripening process.

**WAYS TO ENJOY**

Move over avocado toast and guacamole! Add avocados to smoothies and puddings to enhance creaminess and satiety. When baking, you can replace butter with avocado in a 1:1 ratio. If a recipe calls for 1 cup of butter, use 1 cup of pureed avocado for a heart-healthy, nutrient-dense alternative.

# OLIVES

## The change that occurs inside the chrysalis is gradual and slow.

First, the caterpillar releases enzymes that digest its own body. Then, it becomes liquid and soupy, leaving only imaginal discs. These discs act as blueprints for the new parts of the butterfly to be created. Caterpillars are born with everything they need to become butterflies.

Perhaps you're inside your own chrysalis. Things may feel confusing, formless, and dark. Trust that you were born with everything you need to metamorphose into your potential. The blueprint for your life and purpose is already within you. With patience and time, OLIVE your dreams can become fully realized.

| | |
|---|---|
| **FUN FACTS** | The first eye shadow in ancient Greece was created by mixing olive oil and charcoal. Olives are an excellent source of oleic acid, a type of monounsaturated fatty acid. Olive oil has been shown to reduce inflammation, decrease the risk of heart disease, protect against Alzheimer's disease, and increase lifespan. Speaking of longevity, the oldest olive tree in the world is in Crete and still produces fruit after 3,000 years! |
| **WAYS TO ENJOY** | Add olives to pizza, salads, or nourish bowls to enhance umami flavor. Spread olive tapenade on bread or crackers, or add to stuffed portobello mushrooms. Olives also make an easy and delicious snack just by themselves. |

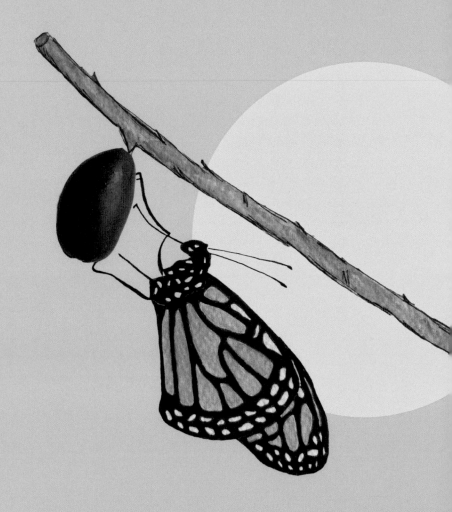

# COMPLEX CARBS

A POEM ABOUT

# COMPLEX CARBS

SWEET POTATOES

BLACK RICE

DELICATA SQUASH

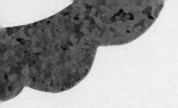

**A POEM ABOUT**

# COMPLEX CARBS

There are two types of carbohydrates —
refined and complex.
When we compare them to each other,
they have very different specs!

'Refined' is processed and has little nutrition,
while 'complex' means it's whole —
the latter contains fiber
which helps us feel more full.

If you're desiring sustained energy
evenly spread throughout the day,
choose complex carbohydrates
to fuel work and play.

They contain vitamins and minerals
and take longer to digest,
replenishing muscle glycogen,
so you're ready for your next quest!

Corn, squash, potatoes,
oats, and brown rice,
all help to balance blood sugar levels
so we tend to act more nice.

Including complex carbohydrates
can help you feel full and strong,
enabling you to enjoy
your activities all day long!

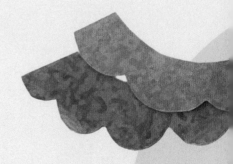

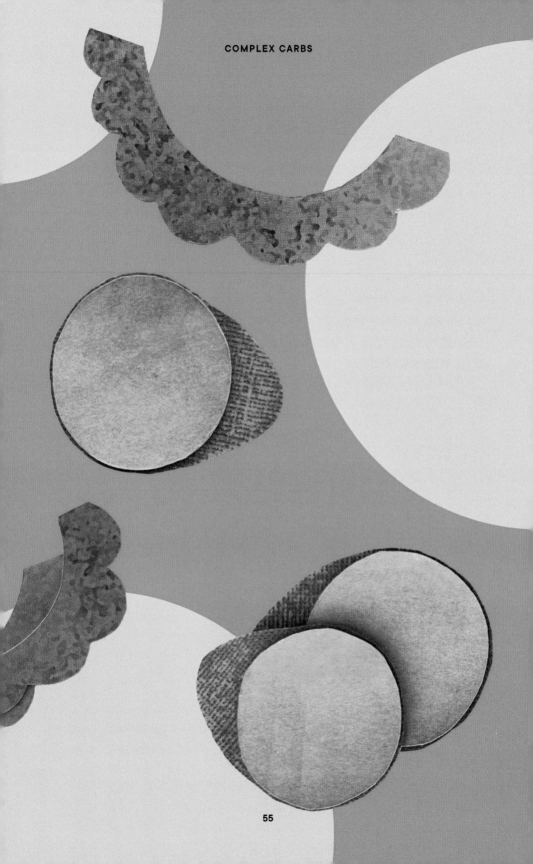

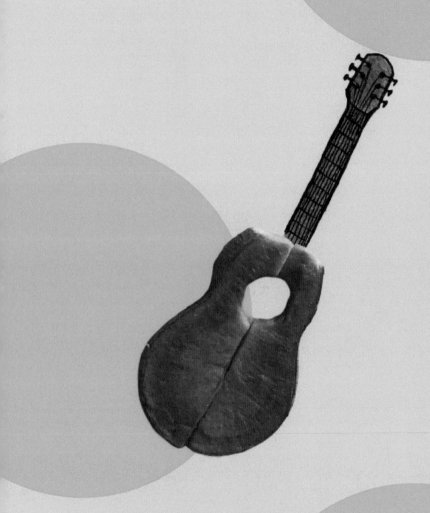

# SWEET POTATOES

Whenever I hear the song "You Can Call Me Al" by Paul Simon, I'm immediately transported back to childhood road trips. Packed in the back of our family's red Honda Accord with camping gear and snacks, my sister and I sang those lyrics along with my parents. Surrounded by the Great Plains and expansive skies, I felt carefree and connected to nature and my family. Those precious memories are awakened by simply hearing a song.

Just as a sweet melody can raise your spirit and invoke positive memories, sweet potatoes contain healthy complex carbohydrates that energize your body and uplift your mood. Additionally, the carbohydrates in sweet potatoes assist with serotonin production, the feel-good neurotransmitter that stabilizes mood and improves feelings of well-being.

**FUN FACTS**

Move over Valentine's Day! February is National Sweet Potato Month. Rich in beta-carotene, fiber, antioxidants, and potassium, sweet potatoes promote heart health and lower LDL cholesterol. Compared to bananas, 1 cup of boiled sweet potatoes contains 1.5 times more potassium. The best place to store them is in a cool, dry, and dark area.

---

**WAYS TO ENJOY**

In the mood for fries? Air-fry sweet potatoes for a colorful and fiber-rich boost of energy and beta-carotene. Going for a long bike ride or hike? Bake them whole, slice them in half, and sprinkle in a little sea salt for a natural, whole food, potassium, and sodium electrolyte replacement. Sweet potatoes make great portable snacks that transport well in backpacks or cycling jerseys to keep you well-fueled and energized to enjoy your favorite activities.

# BLACK RICE

Life is like a piano. The white keys are happy moments, and the black keys are the sad ones. Both are needed to make beautiful music and a beautiful life.

**FUN FACTS**

Black rice gets its purple color from anthocyanin, a powerful antioxidant that fights inflammation. It is also known as "forbidden rice" because it was considered so nutritious and medicinal in ancient China that it was reserved exclusively for royalty. It has a nutty flavor, is a good source of iron, and contains more protein than white and brown rice.

---

**WAYS TO ENJOY**

Use black rice as a nutrient-dense, gluten-free base for grain bowls, rice pudding, and stir-fries. Sprinkle black rice into salads or pair with your favorite curry for a pop of color and chewy texture.

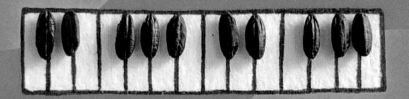

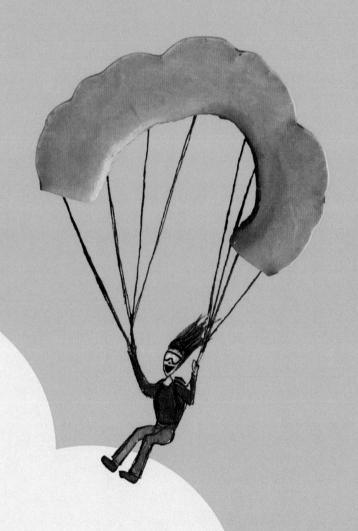

# DELICATA SQUASH

Instead of ignoring or SQUASHing your fears before taking a big leap, try writing them down. Describe the worst-case scenario that could happen if you were to make that jump. Then objectively examine it. Often our worst fears are much scarier in our heads than on paper. Usually, what we fear the most is what we most need to do.

One of the scariest things I did was quit my full-time clinical nutrition job of 11 years to start my private practice. My old job offered a stable income and health insurance. But I wasn't fulfilled. So, I sat and wrote all my fears down. I looked at them, created a plan, budgeted for my decision, and then bravely took the leap.

I didn't ethereally coast over clouds in a state of bliss. Instead, I worked harder than I'd worked before. But I've never looked back, and making that leap catapulted me on an exciting, fulfilling, and remarkable ride that I might have missed if I stayed comfortable and safe on the ground.

**FUN FACTS**

Delicata squash was first introduced in 1894 by Peter Henderson Company of New York. It was popular until the Great Depression when its thin skin made it difficult to be stored or transported long distances. It was not until the 1990s, when a new and improved variety of Delicata, known as the Cornell Bush, was bred, that it began to grow in popularity as a favored winter squash in the United States.

---

**WAYS TO ENJOY**

As its name suggests, Delicata squash has a delicate, thin, edible rind. It can be roasted, sautéed, baked, or stuffed. Additionally, you can toast and season its seeds for a crunchy and delicious snack.

# HERBS & SPICES

# HERBS & SPICES

---

## CHIVES

---

## DILL/THYME

---

## BLACK PEPPER

---

## CALENDULA

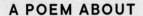

## A POEM ABOUT
# HERBS & SPICES

Herbs and spices, flavor and season,
offer other benefits too —
they're anti-inflammatory and anti-cancer,
they support cognition and mood.

You can easily grow them at home
in your garden or window sill.
They're power-packed, small but mighty,
impacting how you feel.

Garlic boosts your immune system,
so if you're coming down with the flu,
add garlic cloves into your soup,
and soon you'll feel brand new!

If you suffer from motion sickness
or have a slightly queasy tummy,
harness the power of ginger
to soothe you while tasting yummy.

Mint, basil, dill, and chives,
there's so many from to choose!
Add them to your salads,
dressings, nourish bowls, and stews.

Each herb and spice
supports body, spirit, and mind.
Similar to you —
they're unique, one-of-a-kind!

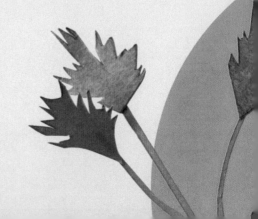

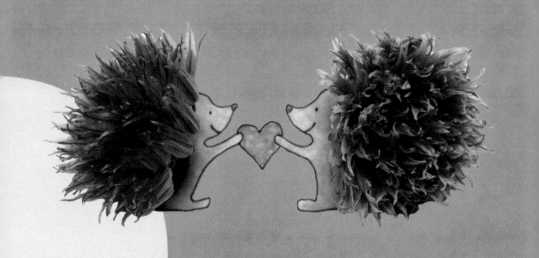

# CHIVES

## We blossom and thrive together in community.

Spending time with loved ones benefits our overall physical and mental well-being. Research shows that people who have loving social connections have stronger immune systems and live longer.

Here are some questions to foster deeper connections:

- What are you currently curious or excited about?
- What advice or wisdom would you offer to your younger self?
- What are some positive ways you've grown since last year?
- What contributions have you made to your family, friends, or community that you're most proud of?

**FUN FACTS**

Chive stalks were used by Romanian gypsies over a century ago as part of their fortune-telling rituals. They would spread them out over a hard surface, and the configuration of the chive bunch would be used to predict the future. In Medieval Ages, chives were hung over doors to ward off evil. Nutritionally, chives contain allyl sulfides that can aid digestion, support heart health, and lower blood pressure.

**WAYS TO ENJOY**

The edible purple blossoms can be added to salads for a vibrant garnish and used to flavor vinegar. Add chive stalks to spice up your homemade green goddess dressing, or sprinkle on salads, toast, soups, or baked potatoes.

# DILL&THYME

## There is pure DILLight in spending quality THYME in nature.

Build a campfire. Stare up into the night sky. Be mesmerized by all the stars. Listen to the sounds of crickets and frogs as dusk settles. Smell the pine needles and redwoods and crisp fresh air. Feel intimately connected to the earth, sky, and mountains. Listen to their poems and songs.

**FUN FACTS**

Dill's name originates from the old Norse word Dilla which means "to lull." It was traditionally used to relieve indigestion and help with insomnia. Hippocrates, the father of medicine, created a mouthwash recipe using dill because of its medicinal properties. For centuries, thyme has been associated with courage, strength, and bravery. Ancient Greeks sprinkled thyme in their baths as a sign of refinement and elegance.

---

**WAYS TO ENJOY**

Add dill to dips and salad dressings, or sprinkle on potato salad. Make your own immune-boosting thyme tea by steeping the leaves in hot water for 10 minutes. Add thyme to season marinades and your favorite pasta dishes.

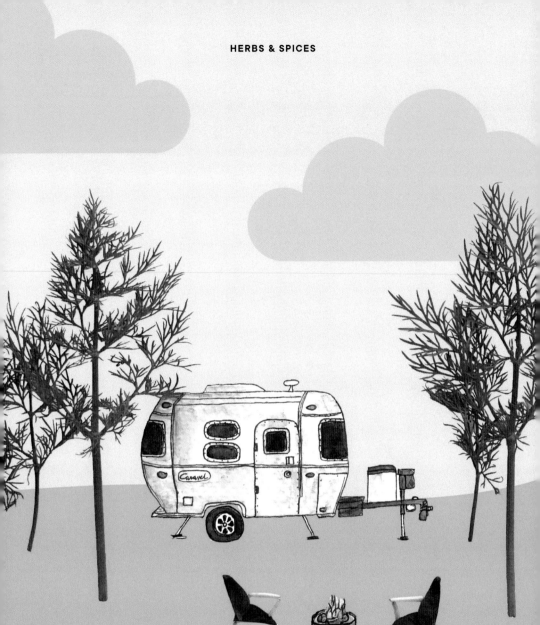

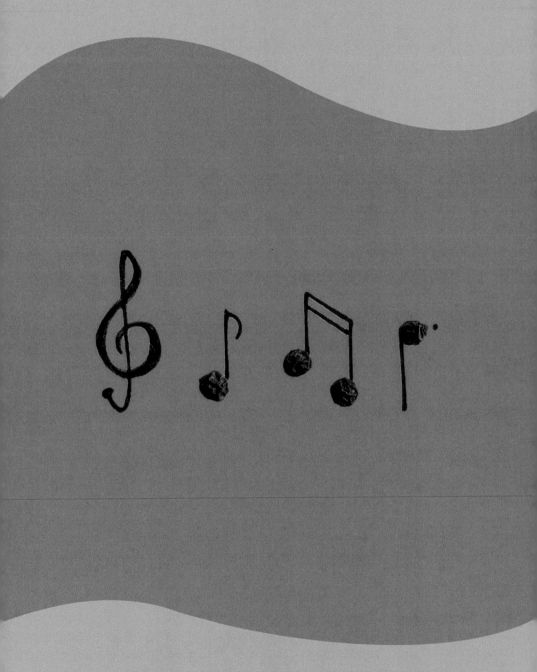

# BLACK PEPPER

When I play Bach on the piano, I'm fascinated by how each hand independently holds its own melody. But together, the fusion of both right and left-hand melodies creates a dynamic synergy of music.

Relationships are also like that. Ideally, each person is grounded in their own uniqueness and independence. When they unite, they're a magical force that co-creates in a powerful way that cannot be done alone.

Who are the people you want to make beautiful music with? We each have a melody to share. Collaborate with the right people. Fuse gifts, talents, and melodies. Birth a new song into the world that makes your heart sing.

**FUN FACTS**

Black pepper and turmeric make a great pair. Piperine, a bioactive compound in black pepper, increases the bioavailability of circumin, the active compound in turmeric by 2000%.

---

**WAYS TO ENJOY**

Curry dishes and soups are delicious opportunities to add turmeric and black pepper. Use them to flavor your next tofu scramble. Enjoy golden turmeric milk as an anti-inflammatory beverage; add some black pepper to increase serum levels and absorption.

# CALENDULA

CALENDULA imagine winning a goldfish at a carnival when you're six and it being your beloved pet for eight years? Usually, when you win a goldfish at a carnival, it lives only a few days. Jostled around in a plastic bag sealed with a tiny rubber band doesn't set the stage for a long and healthy life. I named her Rainbow, and she was my first pet. I fed her fish flakes, regularly cleaned her bowl, bought her fresh aquarium plants with sea snails, and talked to her.

I loved her, knowing she beat the odds. Some friendships are similar. The ones formed randomly at a party, on a walk, or sitting next to each other at a cafe. The chances of making a lasting connection were as slim as a ping-pong ball finding its way into a glass bowl, but they lasted. And I cherish them all, knowing they miraculously beat the odds.

**FUN FACTS**

Calendula symbolizes fire and sunshine with its bright orange and yellow petals. They're often used in Indian wedding bouquets and decorations to symbolize passion and fertility for the newlyweds. In traditional herbal medicine, calendula flowers promote wound healing, and are used to treat eczema, burns, insect bites, headaches, and stomach ailments.

---

**WAYS TO ENJOY**

Calendula petals can be eaten raw or cooked. Add them to salads, salsas, rice dishes, and scrambles. Dried calendula can be substituted for saffron with its tangy and peppery taste. Or, enjoy this vibrant flower in non-food products like soap, body scrub, or oil form to help improve and soothe skin.

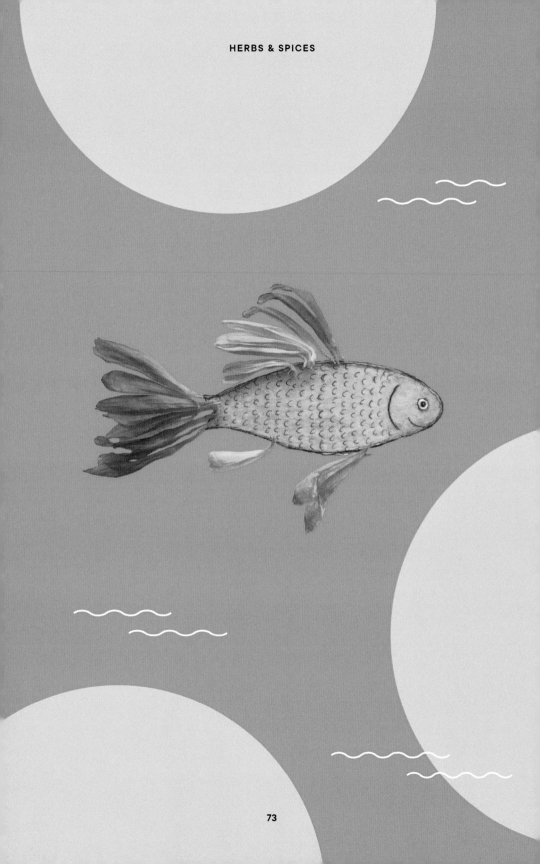

# *the* GRATITUDE BOWL

**TO CATHERINE MADDEN,** for infusing my life
with inspiration and childlike joy.

**TO RINA MARFATIA AND DANIELLE CORREA,**
for being my mycelium network of creativity.

**TO DAD AND MOM,** for encouraging and
enhancing my creative spirit with your unconditional
love, field trips, and generous resources.

**TO PRAVEENA KUMAR,** for your steady,
sustained support throughout the years.

**TO THE TEAM AT FLIGHT DESIGN CO.
AND ALI LAWRENCE,** for providing support,
structure, and editorial guidance.

**TO MATTHEW MEIKLE,** for helping me
combine everything together and bringing my
vision to life with your talent and graphic design.

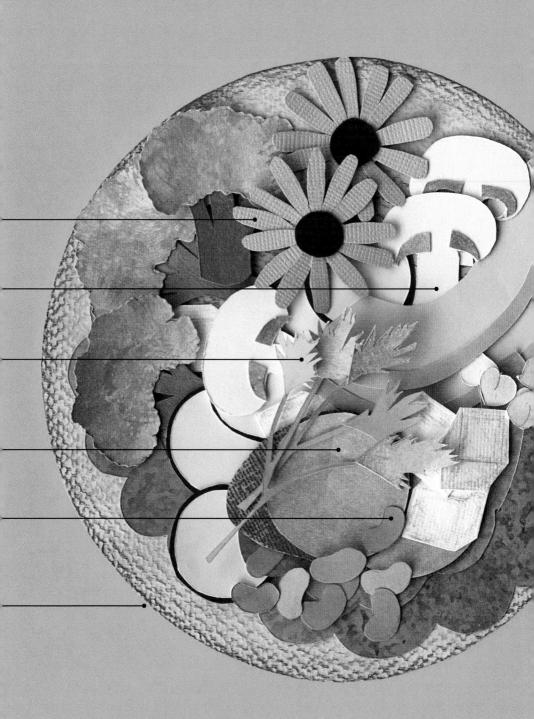

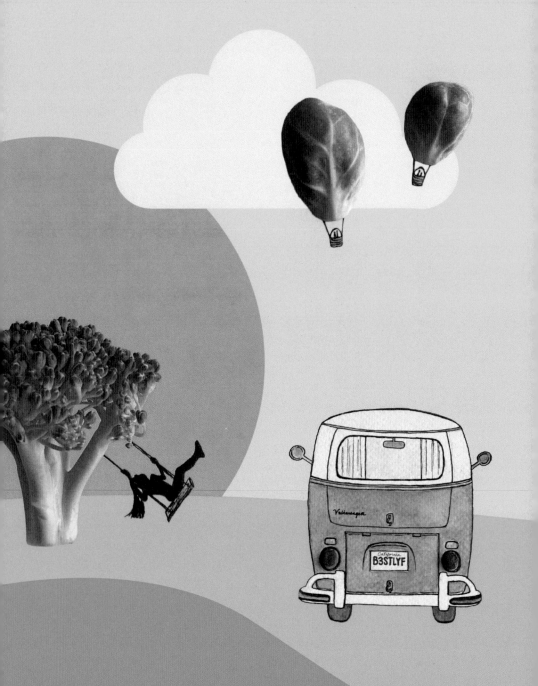

Made in the USA
Monee, IL
18 July 2024

07cd07f2-ff3c-4164-a6d9-195f7f8ea62cR01